Edilaine Soares dos Santos

Epidemiological Survey in the Municipality of Penedo-AL

Edilaine Soares dos Santos

Epidemiological Survey in the Municipality of Penedo-AL

Its importance for the organization of oral health services

ScienciaScripts

Imprint

Any brand names and product names mentioned in this book are subject to trademark, brand or patent protection and are trademarks or registered trademarks of their respective holders. The use of brand names, product names, common names, trade names, product descriptions etc. even without a particular marking in this work is in no way to be construed to mean that such names may be regarded as unrestricted in respect of trademark and brand protection legislation and could thus be used by anyone.

Cover image: www.ingimage.com

This book is a translation from the original published under ISBN 978-613-9-63174-2.

Publisher:
Sciencia Scripts
is a trademark of
Dodo Books Indian Ocean Ltd. and OmniScriptum S.R.L publishing group

120 High Road, East Finchley, London, N2 9ED, United Kingdom
Str. Armeneasca 28/1, office 1, Chisinau MD-2012, Republic of Moldova, Europe
Printed at: see last page
ISBN: 978-620-7-77158-5

SUMMARY

DESIGN

This research consisted of a cross-sectional observational epidemiological study, which aimed to assess the individual risk of dental caries and risk factors related to oral cancer in different areas of the same municipality in different age groups: 0-2, 2-9, 10-19, 20-59 and over 60 years. The aim was to draw up an intervention plan based on promotion, prevention, access and prioritization of dental care. For this purpose, we used a form proposed by the Management of the Oral Health Unit of the Alagoas State Health Department in 2016, contained in the "Manual for Basic Oral Health Care in the State of Alagoas".

SUMMARY

Epidemiological surveys are important for knowing the prevalence of oral diseases and thus planning, implementing and evaluating health actions. This study was therefore carried out in order to verify the prevalence of dental caries and risk factors for oral cancer among different age groups and to assess the needs for oral health care, actions and promotion in two Family Health Strategy teams in the municipality of Penedo-AL. A cross-sectional study was carried out with 1.885 rural (868) and urban (1011) residents aged 0-2, 2-9, 10-19, 20-59 and +60 years were classified by 9 dentists, previously trained and calibrated, as to their risk of tooth decay: 1 (low); 2 (medium); 3 (high) and contributing factors to oral cancer: alcoholism, smoking, use of ill-fitting dentures and mucosal alterations. The data was submitted to descriptive analysis and Kappa with intra- and inter-examiner agreement of 100% and 95%, respectively. Overall, there were more risk 1 and 2 individuals in the urban area (393 and 441, respectively) than in the rural area (262 and 234). However, the rural area (372) had twice as many risk 3 individuals as the urban area (177). In the 0-2 age group, there were no differences between urban and rural areas, regardless of the risk of tooth decay. Prevalence of tooth decay was different in the regions studied, with the urban area standing out in terms of low risk. With regard to risk factors for oral cancer, the prevalence of smoking and alcohol consumption was very similar between the two regions. However, this was not the case for the use of dentures, with the rural area (152) standing out compared to the urban area (87) in the 20-59 age group. The prevalence of mucosal alterations in the same age group (20-59 years) was also a relevant factor between the two regions, with the rural area (32) having twice as many mucosal alterations as the urban area (15). These results suggest oral health promotion and prevention, improved access to dental services and the need to extend risk factor control actions to the younger population.

Key words: Epidemiology. Dental caries. Oral cancer

1. INTRODUCTION

From a national perspective, the most important oral problems in public health are: dental caries, periodontal disease, malocclusions, oral cancer and cleft lip and palate. Of these pathologies, dental caries and periodontal disease, despite the epidemiological changes that have taken place in recent years, are still the most prevalent dental problems, affecting between 50% and 99% of people in most communities (Brasil, 2010). In addition, INCA estimates for Brazil in 2012 predicted that there would be 14,170 new cases of oral cancer, of which 9,990 would occur in men and 4,180 in women (INCA, 2013). Given this situation, it can also be considered a public health problem due to its high prevalence in the population, its strong impact on individuals and society (from an economic point of view), the fact that it can be prevented and the fact that effective treatment is available (Gjermo et al., 2002).

Dental caries is defined as a chronic disease resulting from a bacterial process that gradually dissolves the outer, more resistant surface of the tooth (enamel) and advances into its interior (dentin and cementum). When this process is not interrupted, the tooth can become so compromised that its presence in the mouth is no longer possible (Thylstrup, 1995). Nevertheless, caries results from a relationship between dental plaque, multiple biological determinants and confounding factors of the disease (socio-economic, behavioral and educational level). The biological determinants are the same in all populations, while the confounding factors do not always influence the dynamics of the disease in the same way (Fejerskov, 1997).

Oral cancer encompasses tissue growths that affect the lips and the interior of the oral cavity, such as the gums, jugal mucosa, hard palate, tongue and lip. There are several factors that can predispose to the development of oral cancer. In addition to host-related factors (age, gender, race, genetic inheritance, nutritional status and general health), there are extrinsic factors such as consumption (food, medication), the occupational environment (the action of chemicals), the cultural environment (lifestyle and habits such as tobacco and alcohol), as well as socioeconomic factors (income, housing, schooling) (Neville, 2016). Other emerging risk factors have been mentioned in the literature, such as chronic irritation of the oral mucosa (Mateus, 2008; Piemonte et al., 2010).

Around 10% of all malignant tumors in the body occur in the mouth. It is estimated that around 7% of the world's population is affected, with India taking first place. In northern Europe and the United States, population screening programs have managed to diagnose 85% of lesions in the pre-malignant stage, preventing progression, although mortality rates have not yet been reduced. In Brazil, late diagnosis means that oral cancer ranks 5th among men and 7th among women in terms of mortality (Brasil, 2012).

Thus, since 1986, the Ministry of Health (MoH) has shown the importance of epidemiological surveys in designing actions to combat oral diseases and access to services. When it carried out the first nationwide epidemiological survey in the area of oral health, in urban areas of 16 state capitals, representative of the five Brazilian regions. The survey of children, adolescents, adults and the elderly aimed to obtain data on dental caries, periodontal disease and access to services (Brasil, 1986). Ten years later, in 1996, the second epidemiological survey was carried out in the 27 Brazilian capitals, in the population aged between 6 and 12, generating data on dental caries (Brasil, 1996). In 2000, the Ministry of Health (MS) began discussing a broad epidemiological survey project that would assess the main health problems in different age groups and include both urban and rural populations.

According to Aerts (2004), the frequency of epidemiological surveys should take into account local differences. At municipal level, surveys should be carried out every 10 years, but this frequency can be reduced in other territorial areas, such as neighborhoods and health districts, depending on the epidemiological profile and the needs of the population.

Thus, certain criteria must be followed in epidemiological surveys so that there is methodological uniformity in the procedures, including the choice of the study sample, the evaluation criteria, the calibration of the examiners, the instruments used and the presentation of the data, so as to enable reproducibility, validity and reliability under the same conditions, in any situation or place. The information generated in these studies allows comparisons to be made over time and space, as well as evaluations of the impact of risk factors and health programs related to health problems (Brasil, 2004).

In this context, Law 8080 of 1990, in its chapter II, article 7, states that, in the development of health actions and services, there should be "the use of epidemiology to establish priorities, allocate resources and guide programs" (Goldbaum, 1996). Thus, surveys serve as important tools for defining, implementing and evaluating collective and individual, preventive and care actions, and should not be an end in themselves, but a way of getting to know the epidemiological reality of a given population, and should be carried out periodically (Antunes, Peres, 2013).

Thus, conducting an epidemiological survey in the municipality of Penedo- AL based on oral health conditions in different areas of the same municipality is essential in order to fulfill one of the principles of the SUS, such as universality and equity, requiring oral health teams to know their local reality and their community. Hence the need to organize actions using programming strategies that use criteria for prioritizing the population most in need, planning promotion, prevention and rehabilitation actions in oral health. Sharing results and priorities with the community in order to achieve social control, so that everyone benefits.

The aim of this study is to demonstrate the importance of an epidemiological survey, based on the risk of tooth decay and knowledge of the local situation, in two neighborhoods with different locations, rural and urban, in the age groups of 0-2, 02-09, 10-19, 20-59, and over 60, as well as to actively search for risk factors for the development of oral cancer in the population. Carried out by the Oral Health team of the Family Health Strategy of the Municipality of Penedo, in order to draw up a prioritization, control, promotion and prevention program based on the profile and age group of this population.

2. BACKGROUND

Following the creation of the family health strategy, a milestone in the decentralization of health management and the inclusion of oral health teams, municipalities have reorganized themselves financially and administratively and various transformations have taken place in relation to their management. One of these transformations concerns the need to know the reality and territorial particularities.

Epidemiological surveys of risk factors for tooth decay and the development of oral cancer are essential strategies for transforming local realities. However, professionals and managers are reluctant to use this tool when it comes to making health decisions. This can be explained by a lack of methodological, technical and organizational knowledge when it comes to planning an epidemiological survey and especially when it comes to working with the data collected. In addition, in the work process of the OHT, care is still strongly geared towards the curative model and there is often no dialogue with the situational diagnosis of the territory to which the OHT is inserted. Decision-making is based solely on subjective criteria at state or federal level, or on poorly developed information which, with the right techniques and data, could provide much more than just information on prevalence or incidence.

CONTRIBUTES

The research therefore aims to collaborate with the process of obtaining data aimed at understanding the reality of oral health, based on an epidemiological survey of risk factors for tooth decay and the development of oral cancer, providing up-to-date data to support the Municipal Health Department in order to qualify the planning of actions, or even point to the focus of the problem rather than palliatively treating its symptoms.

3. LITERATURE REVIEW

3.1 Epidemiology and dental caries

The health literature has historically emphasized almost exclusively the study of diseases and their correlates (Coelho et al., 2002), a fact that is generated by the inability to define the object of health (Almeida Filho, 2000; 2006). Although intellectual efforts towards a positive conceptualization of health are already evident, such as the ecosystem approach (Minayo, 2002) and the salutogenic model (AntonovskY, 1996), this discussion has not yet been consistently incorporated into the field of public health and, consequently, epidemiology (Ayres, 2002).

Most research in the field of epidemiology has focused on the study of risk factors. The epidemiological risk paradigm, also known as the "black box" paradigm (Susser & Susser, 1996), came to the fore in the second half of the 20th century with the increase in mortality from chronic non-communicable diseases (Barata, 2005). The term "risk factors" is used to designate quantified probabilities of individual susceptibility to negative events (Jessor et al., 1995) or damage (Almeida Filho, Coutinho, 2007) to health and well-being.

Oral health epidemiology is defined as studies that provide basic information on the oral health and/or dental treatment needs of a population at a given time and place. Its main objectives are to understand the importance of dental problems and to monitor changes in disease levels and patterns over time (Antunes, Peres, 2013).

In Brazil, almost 27% of children aged 18 to 36 months and 60% of children aged 5 years have at least one deciduous tooth with decay. In the permanent dentition, almost 70% of 12-year-olds and around 90% of adolescents aged 15 to 19 have at least one permanent tooth with decay. Among adults and the elderly, the situation is even more serious: the average number of decayed teeth among adults (35 to 44 years old) is 20.1 teeth and 27.8 teeth in the 65 to 74 age group. Analysis of this data also points to progressive and early tooth loss: more than 28% of adults and 75% of the elderly have no functional teeth in at least one arch (BRASIL, 2003).

Carious lesions are considered to be the clinical manifestation of a bacterial infection. The metabolic activity of bacteria results in a continuous process of demineralization and remineralization of dental tissue, and an imbalance in this process can cause a progression of demineralization of the tooth with the consequent formation of a carious lesion. This process is influenced by many determining factors, which makes dental caries a multifactorial disease. It is now considered that the earlier stages of the disease before the cavity can be halted by health promotion and prevention actions. Therefore, restorative treatment of the cavity alone does not guarantee control of the disease process, and it is also necessary to intervene in its determinants in order to prevent new cavities and recurrences in restorations (Brasil, 2008).

It is of the utmost importance that epidemiological data be used to support the planning of oral health actions for the population, so that the intervention can result in the necessary impact to control oral diseases, promote health and improve quality of life, analyzing the reality of the area of coverage, through a comparison between the local situation and the goals proposed by the World Health Organization (WHO) and other national studies (Chaves and Silva, 2007).

In the field of public policy, health promotion represents a promising strategy for tackling and resolving the health problems that affect human populations and their surroundings (Buss, 2000). With the new health policy, created through the introduction of the Family Health Programme (PSF) in 1994, which was established as a priority strategy for organizing primary care according to the precepts of the SUS. It should be guided by the following principles: First contact, longitudinality, comprehensiveness, coordination, family approach and community focus (Starfield, 2002).

In the area of oral health, the expansion of care and access to comprehensive actions for the individual and their family was established by the inclusion of Oral Health Teams (ESB) in the Family Health Strategy (ESF), through Ordinance GM/MS 1.444 of December 28, 2000, which determined the financial incentive for reorganizing oral health care provided to municipalities. The norms and guidelines for this were regulated by Ministerial Order GM/MS No. 267 of March 6, 2001. As of decree no. 673 of 2003, the Ministry of Health began to fund the ESBs in a 1:1 ratio to the Family Health Strategy (ESF) teams. In the ESF model, the family is the protagonist of disease prevention and control actions and must be monitored by the teams. However, Law 8080 of 1990, in its chapter II, article 7, states that, in the development of health actions and services, there must be "the use of epidemiology to establish priorities, allocate resources and guide programming" (Goldbaum, 1996).

Thus, in 2003, the Ministry of Health, in partnership with Brazilian health departments, universities and organizations, concluded the National Oral Health Survey (Brazil, 2004).

In this survey, 108,921 people were examined in the 5 Brazilian macro-regions in 250 randomly selected municipalities (50 in each macro-region), which showed a picture of oral health conditions in Brazil (Roncali, et al., 2000). The results of this survey guided a National Oral Health Policy (Costa et al., 2006).

Studies carried out in the 1980s found a higher prevalence of dental caries in the rural population compared to the urban population (Marques et al., 1986). In the 1990s, there was a reduction in tooth decay in rural areas, but recent studies suggest that oral health in rural populations is still quite precarious (Abreu et al., 2004). And that social deprivation seems to be related to the experience and severity of dental caries in adolescents in the state of São Paulo (Gushi et al., 2010).

With a view to planning oral health actions at the Barâo Geraldo Health Center, in the municipality of Campinas (SP), an epidemiological survey was carried out in 2003 in two public schools, located in the urban and rural areas of the same municipality, in order to observe the prevalence of tooth decay and assess treatment needs and access to dental care. At this point, there was a disparity between the prevalence of cavities in the two populations, where the DMFT at 12 years of age for the rural school was 3.0 and for the urban school it was 0.87, prompting the local manager to set up a dental clinic in the rural area, as the lack of one in the family health center made it difficult for that population to access dental care.

In a study carried out in the municipality of Pindoba-AL in 2016 in schools located in rural areas, based on the risk index for dental caries (risk 1, 2, 3) and periodontal disease, the need to use dentures. The aim was to draw up an intervention plan for dental prevention and treatment for students with any oral health problems. A percentage of 26.6% to 52.17% of the number of schoolchildren with risk 3 was found (Omena, 2016).

Freysleben et al. (2000), emphasize the importance of knowing oral health conditions and planning dental actions that ensure health promotion and early intervention, given that caries is a complex and multifactorial problem with population characteristics and is still considered one of the main oral health problems (Costa et al., 2013).

A study carried out by Mialhe et al. (2008) on the oral health knowledge of the population and the importance of the health team in educational practices, in which they evaluated 114 individuals aged between 15 and 65 years. When asked about the concept of dental caries, the majority of answers (26.3%) were that caries means bacteria on the teeth; 44%

answered that lack of oral hygiene is what causes dental caries and the majority (78.9%) had no knowledge of periodontal diseases. A large proportion of individuals (42.1%) reported not having access to information about oral health, despite 71% using private clinics as their dental service. The results showed some variations in people's perceptions of the etiology and clinical manifestations of the main oral diseases, with the majority of interviewees having some knowledge of these problems, highlighting the importance of the health team in helping the population to control oral diseases and build healthy attitudes and environments.

3.2 Oral Cancer and Risk Factors

Oral cancer is the eighth most common type of cancer in the world, affecting around 7% of the world's population (Massano et al., 2006). In Brazil, this type of cancer corresponds to the 7th highest incidence of all cancers, ranking 5th among men and 12th among women (INCA, 2016). It has become a public health problem due to the large number of patients diagnosed each year and its repercussions on society. INCA estimates for Brazil in 2012 predicted 14,170 new cases of oral cancer, of which 9,990 were expected to occur in men and 4,180 in women (INCA, 2013).

Of all types of oral cancer, around 90% are squamous cell carcinomas. As defined by the World Health Organization (WHO), oral squamous cell carcinoma (OSCC) is characterized by being an invasive epithelial neoplasm with varying degrees of squamous differentiation and a propensity for early lymph node metastasis (Johnson, 2005). The clinical features are quite variable, such as leukoplastic, erythroplastic and leukoerythroplastic aspects, with or without ulcerations and exophytic, endophytic and/or verrucous growth, which is generally asymptomatic, although in more advanced cases pain may occur (Neville, 2016).

The etiology of oral cancer is a sum of carcinogenic factors that can lead to the onset of the disease. The main ones are extrinsic, such as smoking and alcohol, which are responsible for approximately 75% of cases in developed countries. This is in addition to chronic exposure to solar radiation in lipid-related cases. When combined, smoking and alcohol act synergistically, significantly increasing the risk of developing oral cancer (Bagan, 2009). Intrinsic factors such as malnutrition, systemic conditions, age, gender, heredity and oncogenic genes have been reported (Wunsch Filho, 2002; Zair, 2001; Biazevic et al., 2006).

Ogden (2005) described how alcohol acts on the oral mucosa and its association with tobacco use in the etiology of carcinomas. The results showed that alcohol acts on the individual's cells, reducing the size of their cytoplasm and consequently altering DNA profiles. Another way in which alcohol acts on the mucosa is by altering the permeability of the oral mucosa. This would be even greater with an increase in the concentration of alcohol and its association with tobacco.

Oral cancer is generally asymptomatic in its early stages and can mimic common benign conditions of the mouth. Despite the ease with which this tumor can be diagnosed, the existence of well-defined precursor lesions and the risk factors known to be involved in a large number of cases, few results have been obtained with regard to its prevention among the population (Andreotti et al., 2006). In Brazil, the rate of identification of initial malignant lesions in the mouth is very low, corresponding to less than 10% of diagnosed cases (Antunes, et al., 2003).

Oral cancer screening should be an integral part of both medical and dental examinations, as early detection is essential. However, in the majority of cases, it is detected late, when the disease is already considered advanced and has higher mortality rates. Diagnosis at the beginning of the disease and immediate treatment give patients an 80 to 85% chance of a cure, while in the advanced stage, the chance of a cure is reduced by 20 to 25% (Mauricio et al., 2009; Neville et al., 2016).

In 2008, the Brazilian Institute of Geography and Statistics (IBGE), together with the National Cancer Institute (INCA), conducted the most recent survey on smoking in people over 15 years of age. It found that 17.2% of the Brazilian population regularly used tobacco, equivalent to 25 million people. The highest prevalence of smokers was found in the South (19%), and the lowest percentages in the Midwest and Southeast (16.9%).

Dedivits et al. (2004) carried out a study by analyzing the clinical records of patients with squamous cell carcinoma of the mouth (SCC) and oropharynx from the head and neck surgery department of the Ana Costa hospital and the Irmandade da Santa Casa de Misericòrdia do Municipio de Santos - SP. Of these patients, 35% were smokers and 74% were alcoholics. The most common site of lesions was the tongue (51.1%) followed by the floor of the mouth (25.5%).

França et al. (2010) described the clinical results obtained with the oral cancer diagnosis and prevention program at the University of Mato Grosso. The program consisted of lectures and oral assessment of users by undergraduate dental students at the university.

Users filled in a questionnaire with their information and drinking and smoking habits, a dental examination for cavities, the need for dentures and a visual examination to detect lesions in the oral cavity. During the five years of the program, 2,573 were examined and 249 biopsies were taken, diagnosing 13 cases of oral cancer. The authors concluded that prevention and early diagnosis of oral cancer are essential and suggest the implementation of diagnosis and prevention programs in other health services.

Scheufen et al. (2011) evaluated the effectiveness and feasibility of diagnosing oral cancer by examining asymptomatic patients belonging to the risk group for the disease. They identified the populations with the highest concentration of smokers and alcoholics in various sectors of society such as hospitals, support groups and churches. In these places, lectures were given with information about tobacco, alcohol and oral cancer and the importance of performing oral self-examination and maintaining good oral hygiene was discussed.

After the lectures, they carried out an oral examination of those present and those who showed alterations in the mucosa were referred to USP's School of Dentistry for a cytopathological examination or biopsy. The authors concluded that the strategy adopted in the study was effective in detecting key lesions in a risk group.

Prado and Passarelli (2009) cite eight items that would be of fundamental importance to the dental surgeon (DS) when counseling patients and diagnosing oral cancer. Based on these items, the DS would be able to guide his patients, as well as recognize and diagnose oral cancer early. Among the risk factors that should be identified and eliminated, the authors mention smoking - because it causes dryness of the oral mucosa, increases the keratin layer and produces thermal-mechanical trauma; alcohol - whose chronic contact with the jugal mucosa acts as a solvent, slowing down the reaction speed with the organism and producing cell damage. The authors also report the importance of a diet rich in nutrients, especially vitamin A, and advise the use of protection against sun exposure, whose ultra violet radiation is capable of causing cell damage to the epithelium and underlying connective tissue. They also emphasize attention to immunodeficiency, especially due to the presence of the HPV virus. They warn about the importance of biopsying pre-cancerous lesions, which, combined with risk factors, increase the chances of them becoming carcinomas in situ. They emphasize adapting to the oral environment by removing irritants and infectious agents from the oral mucosa and provide guidance on oral self-examination.

Chronic trauma to the oral mucosa is a risk factor that has been widely reported in the literature. It is thought to result from the constant mechanical irritant action of an intra-oral injury agent on the epithelial cells. These agents can be represented by biting of the mucosa, irritation from removable dentures, toothbrush injury, exposure of the mucosa to an acute edge of dental caries or the action of any other external irritant, which can develop into malignancy (Piemonte et al., 2010; Mateus, 2008). Traumatic ulcers mainly affect the jugal mucosa, lips, gums, palate, sulcus floor and tongue. They are easily diagnosed and have a multifactorial etiology (Goiato et al., 2005).

Thus, authors such as Quirino et al. (2006) report that the diagnosis of lesions with cancerous potential is favorable to dental surgeons and the patient themselves, since the mouth is considered to be an easily accessible place where suspicious alterations can be checked through self-examination. However, the population is not informed and neglects signs and symptoms (Cimardi, Fernandes, 2009). This may already be changing, given that after the inclusion of oral health teams (ESB) in the ESF there has been an increase in the number of people receiving dental care, giving the dental surgeon a fundamental role in the prevention and early diagnosis of oral cancer (Brasil, 2008).

3.3 Population unawareness of oral cancer risk factors

Popular health education is an excellent tool for popularizing and disseminating technical and scientific knowledge, bringing the population and professionals closer together and demystifying the disease, which, when brought closer to the population, makes it possible to identify risk factors and seek prevention/diagnosis, although professionals need adequate training (Vidal et al., 20009). However, Antunes et al. (2007); Quirino et al. (2006); Ribeiro et al. (2008), who sought to assess the knowledge and health practices of the adult population about mouth cancer, have in common the low understanding that people, in general, have of this disease. This is related to factors such as the population's lack of knowledge about the tumor, its signs and risk factors, as well as professionals - dentists and doctors - who do not pay attention to or suspect the lesions observed (Tescarollo, Freire, 2018).

A survey of 826 students from public secondary and elementary schools in the Sertâo region (Arcoverde, Caraibas, Venturosa) of Pernambuco, Brazil, found that 60% of this sample said they had heard of the disease; 20% pointed to smoking, alcohol and the sun as risk factors; 96% did not know about self-examination, and 80% said they did not know how to proceed if a lesion was identified (Vidal et al, 2009).

Another study by Zaneti et al. (2011) used retrospective data from questionnaires carried out with 776 people who took part in a health campaign held in the state of São Paulo in 2009. The 17-question questionnaire sought to characterize the study population in terms of knowledge, habits and attitudes, such as: etiological factors; signs and symptoms; prevention; self-examination; and visits to the dentist. The results showed that the average age of the participants was 42 years (SD±10.1) and that they had little schooling (63.1% only had primary education). The majority (64.6%) had not received any advice about mouth cancer, and only 32.1% were able to name some of the probable causes of the disease. Suspicious signs of the disease were reported by 27.6% of people, and only 15.9% said they knew about self-examination of the mouth. In view of the results presented, the authors concluded that it is important to carry out educational campaigns aimed at the prevention and early diagnosis of mouth cancer, as misinformation was high.

Lima et al. (2005), evaluated that it is difficult to improve knowledge about cancer, since people do not see themselves as a population at risk, with an aggravating factor in the case of mouth cancer, since studies (Quirino et al., 2006; Molina et al., 2006) have shown that the Brazilian population has little knowledge that cancer can occur in the mouth and that the disease is mainly linked to the lifestyle of each individual.

Furthermore, according to Matos et al. (2003), there is no point in saying that self-examination is a simple method if the population doesn't have this practice incorporated and that suspicious cancer lesions (changes in color, ulcers, swelling) are difficult to identify, as people more easily perceive the more visible and concrete manifestations that characterize the advanced stages of the disease, such as difficulty chewing, speaking, rapid weight loss or pain.

All of this highlights the importance of carrying out health education programs, encouraging self-examination and measures to combat alcohol and tobacco consumption. Although there is no consensus on the effectiveness of oral cancer screening campaigns, this was confirmed in a study carried out by Kujan et al. (2005) in which they carried out a systematic review of these strategies and concluded that there is not enough evidence to recommend or not to recommend visual examination in the general population.

Apparently, when the screening campaign is aimed at people at high risk of developing the disease, it is effective, as demonstrated by Cruz et al. (2002) in a study of 803 people in the United States. The authors concluded that these programs represent an opportunity not only for early detection of the disease, but also for raising awareness and concern about oral cancer. Gourin et al. (2009), in a screening study with 89 people in Baltimore in the United States, also concluded that there was a breadth of knowledge of the individual, which made it easier to identify people who required more detailed assessment. On the other hand, when the campaign doesn't focus on susceptible groups, it tends to be ineffective, as demonstrated by Antunes et al. (2007), who evaluated the results of the oral cancer prevention and diagnosis campaign carried out in conjunction with the flu vaccination campaign in the state of São Paulo in 2004.

4. OBJECTIVES

GENERAL OBJECTIVE

To demonstrate the importance of the epidemiological survey in the Oral Health Strategy based on the caries risk index and risk factors for the development of oral cancer among different age groups, in order to draw up a program for prioritizing care, control, promotion and prevention based on two teams from different locations in the municipality of Penedo-AL.

SPECIFIC OBJECTIVES

*   Keeping oral health epidemiological data up to date in support of the Municipal Health Department.

*   Organize access to dental services for communities

*   Developing promotion and prevention actions geared to the profile and age group of the population.

*   Making the population co-responsible for caring for their oral health,

including the main causal agents.

5. MATERIALS AND METHODS

5.1 SELECTING THE AREA AND GROUP TO STUDY

Penedo is a municipality with 64,292 inhabitants (IBGE, 2016), located in the southern region of the state of Alagoas, with a population density of 93 inhabitants/km^2 . The Family Health Strategy has 19 oral health teams, 13 of which are located in urban areas and 6 in rural areas. The municipality also has a type 2 Dental Specialty Center (CEO), set up in 2004 after the creation of the National Oral Health Policy (Brasil Sorridente).

In order to carry out this research, it was necessary to select an area and a group to study. In order to meet the objectives of the study, a health unit in an urban location (Vitória) and another in a rural location were randomly selected, all with a full Family Health Strategy team, composed of a doctor, nurse, dentist (CD), oral health assistant (ASB) or oral health technician (TSB), community health agent (ACS) and nursing technician, covering 100% of the population. The urban health unit, Vitória, covers 9 micro-areas and is responsible for approximately 4,000 users. The rural health unit, Capela, located approximately 15km from the city, covers 07 micro-areas, with approximately 3,500 users.

This study was carried out by 9CDs, 9 ASBs and the CHAs responsible for their respective micro-areas. The age groups were chosen in accordance with the recommendations of the Ministry of Health, prioritizing follow-up and possible oral pathologies that may arise during life. The age groups studied were: 0-2 years (babies); 2-9 years (children), 10-19 years (adolescents), 2059 years (adults) and the elderly over 60. For minors, their parents had to sign an informed consent form. **For** those over the age of 18, the parents had to sign the informed consent form. Individuals who did not wish to take part in the study, those who were not at home at the time of the team's visit and those who were bedridden and/or hospitalized were excluded from the intraoral examination.

The 2-9 age group is the ideal age for educational and preventive oral health programs, as well as routine home visits to avoid early extraction of deciduous teeth. In individuals aged 10-19, the adolescent period, it is very common for certain problems to occur, such as bulimia (an eating disorder related to unrestrained eating and then inducing vomiting in order to control weight), which can lead to dental erosion and decay on the lingual face of the front teeth, as well as the use of piercings, which can cause inflammatory and infectious complications. Between the ages of 17 and 21, third molars usually erupt, most of which are difficult to reach and require special care when brushing. At this stage, most of the permanent teeth most at risk of decay have already erupted (Brasil, 2008). Adults in the 20-59 age group, a period in which chronic diseases such as diabetes, tuberculosis, AIDS and others develop, can have oral manifestations. Although these problems occur in other age groups, they are very important in this age group. In the elderly over 60, it is important to observe the intensity of oral diseases, the state of conservation of the teeth and the prevalence of edentulism, which are mainly a reflection of their living conditions and access to oral health actions and services, with a strong social component.

5.2 TYPE OF STUDY

This was a cross-sectional observational study of 1,885 residents. These were from rural (868) and urban (1011) locations in the 0-2, 2-9, 10-19, 20-59 and +60 age groups, who were classified by 9 dentists, previously trained and calibrated, as to their risk of cavities: 1 (low); 2 (medium); 3 (high) (Brazil, 2008) and assessed as to the risk factors for developing oral cancer.

5.3 ETHICAL CONSIDERATIONS

This study was conducted in accordance with the precepts determined by Resolution 196 of 10/10/1996 of the National Health Council of the Ministry of Health after approval by the Ethics Committee of the Sao Leopoldo Mandic Research Center (No. 2.115.933). The study was carried out between June and August 2017, and each clinical examination and form was filled in after signing the Informed Consent Form (ANNEX A-B).

5.4 CALIBRATION

The training and calibration of the examiners took place in the auditorium of the Municipal Health Department. The work team consisted of nine examiners (dentists from the Family Health Strategy) and nine annotators (Oral Health Assistants - OHA) and the Community Health Agents (CHA) from the respective micro-areas. The calibration process adopted the criteria established by SB Brasil 2010 (BRASIL, 2009b).

The survey was carried out in three stages, the first being theoretical training, in which the risk indices and parameters to be surveyed, the instruments to be used and how to fill in the examination form were presented. For the CHAs, this stage was used to approach the user about taking part in the survey. In the second stage, the examiners and note-takers were trained by examining children aged 5-9 and adults aged 20-59, with six children and six adults for training and 10 from each age group for calibration (Brazil, 2001). A duplicate test was carried out on every ten children/adults, and the examiner was not informed of this test so as not to interfere with the reproducibility results. The Kappa test was applied to assess intra- and inter-examiner agreement, and calibration was considered satisfactory only if the disagreement was equal to or lower than that recommended by the World Health Organization (WHO), which considers disagreement to be around 1 to 15% for most assessments (Brazil, 1997). The third stage of the process was a theoretical meeting to discuss the main doubts encountered, as well as to collectively standardize the criteria adopted in the research.

5.5 ASSESSING THE RISK OF DENTAL CARIES AND CONTRIBUTING FACTORS TO ORAL CANCER

The research methodology used for this study to assess the individual risk of dental caries and oral cancer is the one set out in the Ministry of Health's Basic Care Notebook No. 17, which recommends that the establishment of parameters is necessary for organizing health actions and services, promoting more effective management action, guaranteeing directionality in the actions developed and improving planning, allowing monitoring and evaluation and giving health teams a differentiated quality in their work process (Brasil, 2008).

The risk analysis is based on parameters related to oral health care through the individual's life cycle, analyzing babies aged 0-24 months, children aged 2-9 years, adolescents aged 10-19 years, adults aged 20-59 years and the elderly over 60 years. As for the risk of tooth decay, each age group has 3 classifications, with values ranging from 1 to 3, and whenever a child is found to be at risk 3, the child is classified as being at high risk. As for the active search for oral cancer, risk factors for the development of lesions were analyzed, with the exception of the 0-24 month age group. In the other age groups, individuals who smoked (use of pipes, habits of chewing tobacco, cigarettes), drank alcohol, used ill-fitting dentures and mucosal lesions were investigated.

Table 1- Parameters used in the assessment of dental caries risk and active search for oral cancer.

	CODE 1	CODE 2	CODE 3	
Objective examination of the mouth caries	* Absence of caries lesions without biofilm, without gingivitis and/or without active white spots. * Tooth restored,	*one or more cavities with chronic lesions but without biofilm, gingivitis or active white spot and/or stain.	*One or more cavities in an active caries lesion situation *Presence of pain and/or abscess	

	but without gingivitis and/or active white spot	*Absence of carious lesions, but presence of bifilm, gingivitis and/or white spot		
Active search for oral cancer	Smoke	Bebe	Injuries due to ill-fitting prostheses	Mucosal lesions
	Pipe Cigarettes Chewing smoke	More than once a week		Addictions or habits

5.6 INTRA-ORAL EXAMINATION

This examination made it possible to collect data to determine the individual risk of dental caries and contributing factors to the development of oral cancer based on the risk indices described in Table 1. All the diagnostic criteria recommended by the WHO were followed. All the necessary equipment was used, including gloves, masks and wooden spatulas. The examinations were carried out house to house, making the most of the ambient light. Each individual was examined only once, after giving informed consent (figure 1 A-B-C).

Figura 1: Clinical examination by a calibrated dental surgeon

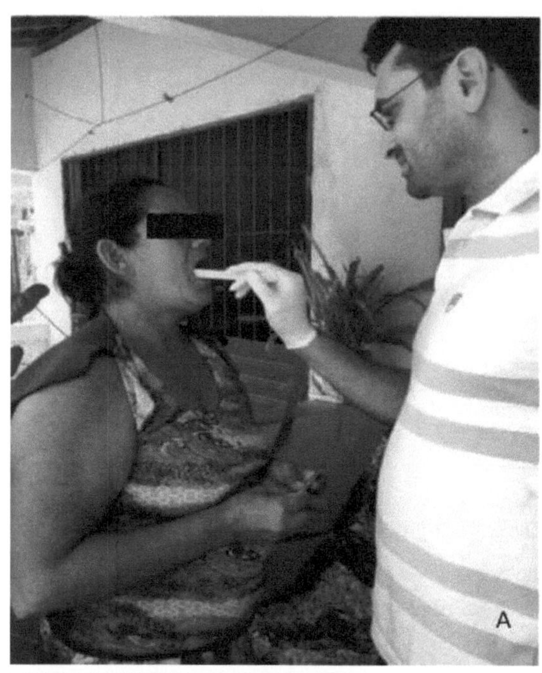
A

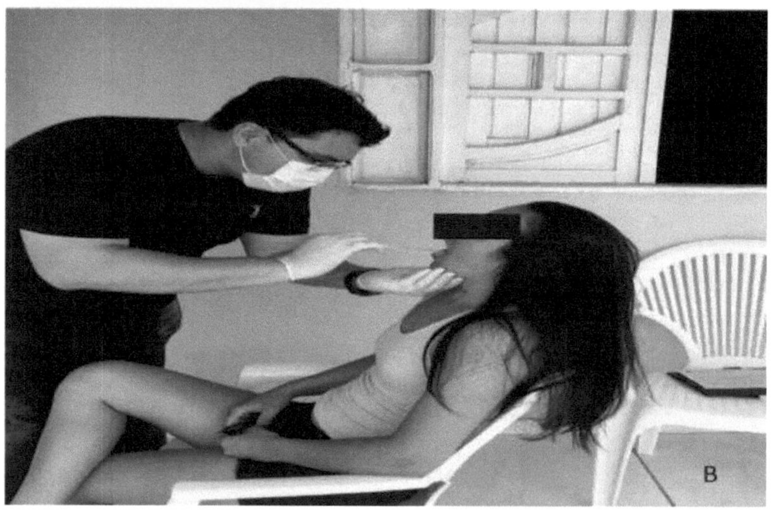
B

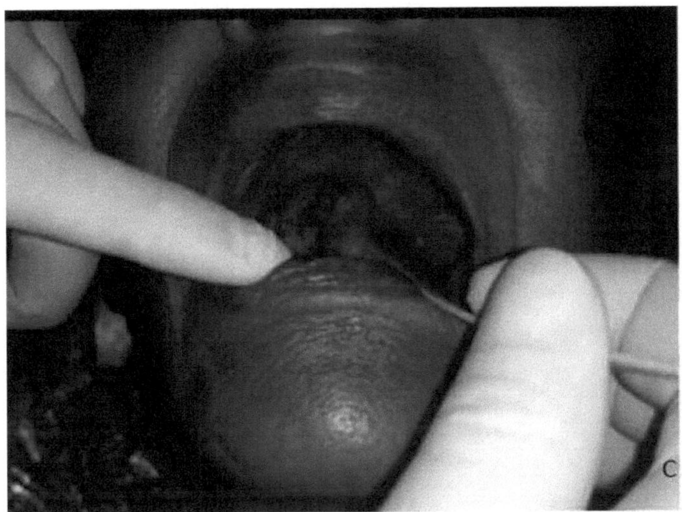

Data collection was carried out by the dental surgeons, oral health assistants and the community health agent responsible for the micro-area. The examinations in each micro-area were carried out by appointment by the CI IA responsible for the area. The examiners went from house to house and while the community health agent introduced the user of their respective micro-area to the dental surgeon for the intra-oral examination, the oral health assistant wrote down the data on a form standardized by the Alagoas state secretariat (figure 1). After carrying out the epidemiological survey, the oral health team met and consolidated the data collected on a specific form.

Figure 1- Form standardized by the Alagoas state secretariat for carrying out epidemiological surveys

EPIDEMIOLOGICAL SURVEY

Need for dental treatment

_______________________________________MunicipalityArea _________________ Micro-areaNº _________ of Family

NAME	Date of Birth	Gender M/F	Code Risto Carie	Periodontal Disease Yes/No	Pregnant women Yes/No	Need for a prosthesis				Active Search for Buccal Cancer				Date	Note
						EratTotal		EratEarcRem							
						Max	Mand	Max	Mand	F	B	P	A		

F=Smokes/ B=Baby/ .P=Wears Prosthesis/ A= Mouth Mucosa Alteration

Figura 2: Consolidated Càrie Risk Sheet

CONSOLIDATED DENTAL CARIES DIAGNOSIS DATA

ÀREANºof Families Registered Nºof Families Visited: Nºof People examined: ___________________

NEED FOR ONTOLOGICAL TREATMENT	AGE RANGE	MICRO AREAS									TOTAL	
		1	2	3	4	5	6	7	S	9	Nº	%
Need for Treatment Code 1 Caries	Oa 24 months											
	02 to Odanos											
	io a 19 a nos											
	20 to 59 years											
	Over 60 to us											
	SUBTOTAL											
	Pregnant women											
Need for Treatment code 2 Caries	O to 24 months											
	02 to 09 to us											
	10 to 19 a nos											
	20 to 59 years											
	Aoma from 60 to											
	SUBTOTAL											
	Pregnant women											
Need for Treatment Code 3 Caries	O to 24 months											
	02 to 09 to us											
	19 years old											
	20 to 59 years old											
	Aoma from 60 to											
	SUBTOTAL											
	Pregnant women											
GRAND TOTAL												

DATE: / ___ / _____   Assi ттatu ra do Responsave I / carl rтtbo

Figura 3: Consolidated oral cancer active search form

CONSOLIDADO DOS DADOS DO DIAGNÓSTICO/ BUSCA ATIVA DO CÂNCER BUCAL

ÁREA:_____________ Nº de Fam. cadastradas______ Nº de Fam. Visitadas:______ Nº de Pessoas examinadas:______

NECESSIDADE DE TRATAMENTO ODONTOLÓGICO	FAIXA ETÁRIA	MICRO-ÁREAS									TOTAL	
		1	2	3	4	5	6	7	8	9	Nº	%
FUMA	02 a 09 anos											
	10 a 19 anos											
	20 a 59 anos											
	Acima de 60 anos											
	SUBTOTAL											
	Gestante											
BEBE	02 a 09 anos											
	10 a 19 anos											
	20 a 59 anos											
	Acima de 60 anos											
	SUBTOTAL											
	Gestante											
USA PRÓTESE	10 a 19 anos											
	20 a 59 anos											
	Acima de 60 anos											
	SUBTOTAL											
	Gestante											
ALTERAÇÃO NA MUCOSA BUCAL	0 a 24 meses											
	02 a 09 anos											
	10 a 19 anos											
	20 a 59 anos											
	Acima de 60 anos											
	SUBTOTAL											
	Gestante											

Município _________________________

DATA: _____/_____/_________

Assinatura do Responsável / carimbo

6. RESULTS

The age of the population examined varied between different age groups, with 1011 located in urban areas and 868 in rural areas.

There were more risk 1 and 2 individuals in the urban area (393 and 441, respectively) than in the rural area (262 and 234). However, the rural area (372) had twice as many risk 3 individuals as the urban area (177), showing very pessimistic results in relation to the team's expectations. Of the 868 individuals assessed in the rural area, only 30% (272) presented risk 1, which meant that they did not need dental treatment.

In the 0-2 age group, there were no differences between urban and rural areas, regardless of the risk of tooth decay. The prevalence of caries was different in the regions studied, with the urban area standing out in terms of low risk, except in the 20-59 age group, where the urban area (287) had twice as many individuals at risk 2 than the rural area (129), presenting at least one cavity with a chronic cavity lesion, or the presence of bifilm, gingivitis and/or white spots, requiring dental treatment and oral health promotion and prevention actions. As illustrated in Table 2.

With regard to the active search for oral cancer in general, similar exposure to smoking and alcoholism was observed for the rural and urban populations. However, this was not the case for the use of ill-fitting prostheses, with the rural area (152) standing out in relation to the urban area (87) in the 20-59 age group. The prevalence of mucosal alterations with malignant potential in the same age group (20-59 years) was also a relevant factor between the two regions, with the rural area (32) having twice as many mucosal alterations as the urban area (15). This suggests the need to intensify and extend actions to control risk factors and broaden access to the younger population. As illustrated in table 3.

Table 2- Dental caries risk index in different age groups of individuals belonging to the ESF health units located in the urban area (PSF Vitória) with 1011 individuals examined and the rural area (PSF Capela), with 868 individuals examined.

Age group	Risk 1		Risk 2		Risk 3	
	Urban	Rural	Urban	Rural	Urban	Rural
0-2 years	21	23	01	01	0	0
2-9 years	63	70	35	47	10	58

10-19 years	84	41	49	24	17	56
25-59 years	149	102	287	129	110	209
Over 60	76	26	69	33	42	49
Total	393	262	441	234	177	372
Percentage	38,8%	30%	43,6%	27%	17,5%	42,8%

Table 3- Risk factors for oral cancer in different age groups of individuals belonging to the ESF health units located in the urban area (PSF Vitória) with 1011 individuals examined and the rural area (PSF Capela) with 868 individuals examined.

| Age group | Urban area | | | | Rural Area | | | |
| | 1011 | | | | 868 | | | |
	Smoke	Bebe	Wears a prosthesis	Mucosal changes	Smoke	Bebe	Wears a prosthesis	Mucosal alteration
2-9 years	02	0	0	01		0	0	
10-19	45	06	0	01	01	04	03	04
20-59	19	94	87	15	53	89	152	32
Over 60	66	22	63	09	32	19	49	16
Total	132	122	150	26	109	112	204	52
Percentage	13%	12%	14,8%	2,5%	12,5%	12,6%	23,5%	5.9%

7. INTERVENTION PLAN

The intervention plan began with a situational diagnosis of the users living in the territory where the ESF vitória and capela health units are located, carried out by the oral health teams through an epidemiological survey.

As discussed above and shown in Table 2, the risk index 3 for users located in the territory of the Capela ESF, in rural areas, was twice as high as that of the Vitória unit, in urban areas. This was due to the difficulty users in micro-areas 5, 6 and 7 had in accessing the health unit and oral health promotion and prevention actions, as well as their low family income. The difficulty of access was mainly associated with location, ranging from 10 to 15 km from the homes of users in the micro-areas mentioned above. In addition, the rural population complained about the absence of health workers in their micro-area and were very unaware of the risk factors for developing oral cancer. Urban dwellers, on the other hand, emphasized the lack of time to go to the health unit during the day. Thus, each population had its own particularities, which meant that the intervention plan proposed by the oral health teams, coordination and management was based not only on the risk indices, but also on the location of the health units and the difficulty of access. As shown in table 1.

Table 1: Intervention plan for rural and urban populations.

Action	Technical and methodological organization of the project
	epidemiological survey
Expected results	Population aware of risk factors for caries and oral cancer; Improvement in caries indices. Community health agents more integrated with oral health teams and the population. The population taking co-responsibility for improving their oral health.
Critical nodes	- Health center far from the micro-areas; - Population with little or no knowledge of the risk factors for developing oral cancer; - People in rural areas work all day. - Age groups between 20-59 resistant to attending the health unit. - Community health agents (ACS) dispersed with the care of their micro area.

	- Families that share toothbrushes, due to low family income.
Actors involved	- Manager - Oral health coordination - Dental surgeon - Oral health assistants - Community Health Agents.
Resources needed	- Structural: Health centers in need of renovation - Financial: Purchase of: Portable or mobile dental clinic, oral hygiene kits; educational material; sunscreen; lip balm; Data Show, television and DVD for waiting rooms. - Political: Provision of funds for the purchase of the above-mentioned items
Strategic action	- Training of CHWs on the importance of their inclusion in the program Oral health promotion, through lectures, educational videos and plays aimed at oral health care and oral self-examination in the micro-area of coverage; - Supervised tooth brushing in the schools covered by the program and quarterly application of fluoride. - Prioritization of dental care for risk 3, making the health agent responsible for the individual's micro area responsible. - In areas where access to the health unit is difficult, the oral health team will go to the user. - Guaranteed lip and sun protection for rural workers; - Creation of the Night Oral Health Program to assist individuals who work during the day. - Guarantee of timely care and transportation to the Dental Specialties Center for treatment not required by the basic health unit (endodontic treatment, gingivectomy, prosthesis, oral and maxillofacial surgery). - Guaranteed consultations with the stomatology specialty for
	users who presented changes in the mucosa with a potential for malignancy. - Intensification of actions in the School Health Program (PSE)

8. FINAL CONSIDERATIONS

The epidemiological survey showed that the risk index for caries disease varied according to age group and location. Individuals in rural areas and in the 25-59 age group were more prone to developing cavities. This suggests that greater attention should be paid to oral health promotion, prevention and treatment.

Epidemiological surveys should be included in the work process of oral health teams and be seen as indispensable for planning, intervention programs and evaluation in the public sector, allowing a proposal for a well-defined local oral health policy.

9. REFERENCES

Abreu MHNG, Pordeus IA, Modena CM. Dental caries among rural schoolchildren in Itaùna (MG), Brazil. Rev Panam Salud Publica. 2004; 16(5): 334-344.

Aerts D, Abegg G, Cesa K. The role of the dental surgeon in the Unified Health System. Cienc. Saud. Colet. 2004;9(1):131-138.

Andreotti M, Rodrigues NA, Cardoso LMN, Figueiredo RAO, Eluf-Neto J, Wünsch- Filho V. Occupation and cancer of the oral cavity and oropharynx. Cad. Saùde Pùblica. 2006; 22(3): 543-552.

Antunes AA, Takano JH, Queiroz TC, Vidal AKL. Epidemiological profile of oral cancer at CEON/HUOC/UPE and HCP. Odontol Clin-Cientif. 2003; 2(3):181-186.

0 Antunes JLF, Toporcov TN, Wunsch-Filho V. Resoluteness of the oral cancer prevention and early diagnosis campaign in Sao Paulo, Brazil. Rev Panam Salud Publica. 2007;21(1):30-36.

Antunes JLF, Peres MA. Epidemiology in Oral Health. 2ª ed. Rio de Janeiro: Guanabara Koogan, 2013.

Ayres, JRCM. Epidemiology, health promotion and the paradox of risk. Revista Brasileira de Epidemiologia.2002;5(1):28-42.

Almeida Filho N. The concept of health: epidemiology's blind spot? Revista Brasileira de Epidemiologia. 2000a; 3(1):4-20.

Almeida FilhoN, Rouquayrol MZ. Introduction to modern epidemiology. 4aed. Rio de Janeiro: Medsi; 2006.

Almeida Filho N, Coutinho D. Causality, contingency, complexity: The future of the concept of risk. PHYSIS: Revista Saùde Coletiva. 2007;17(1):95-137.

Antonovsky A. The salutogenic model as a theory to guide health promotion. Health Promotion International, London. 1996;11(1):11-18.

Barata RB. Social epidemiology. Revista Brasileira de Epidemiologia. 2005;8(1):7- 17.

Brasil. Ministry of Health - National Oral Health Division. Epidemiological survey on oral health: Brazil, urban area. Brasilia; 1986. 137p.

Brazil. Ministry of Health. Health Care Secretariat. Department of Health Care and Promotion. Coordination of Oral Health. Epidemiological Survey of Oral Health: 1st stage - dental caries - project. Brasilia; 1996.

Brazil. Ministry of Health. SB 2000: Oral Health Conditions in the Brazilian Population in 2000. Brasilia; 2000.

Brazil. Ministry of Health. Oral Health Technical Area. SB Brasil 2000 Project - Oral health conditions of the Brazilian population in the year 2000: examiner's manual. Brasilia: Ministry of Health; 2001.

Brazil. Ministry of Health. Health Care Secretariat. Department of Primary Care. National Oral Health Coordination. SB Brazil 2003 Project. Oral Health Conditions of the Brazilian Population, 2002-2003: main results. Brasilia: Ministry of Health; 2004.

Brazil. Ministry of Health. Health Care Secretariat. Department of Primary Care. Oral Health. Series A. Normas e Manuais Técnicos - Caderno de atençâo Bàsica, n°17. 1ª ed. Ministério da Saù; 2008.

Brazil. Ministry of Health. Secretariat of Health Policies. Department of Primary Care. Oral Health Technical Area. SB 2010 Project: oral health conditions of the Brazilian population in 2010. Brasilia: Ministry of Health; 2009.

Brazil. Ministry of Health. National Cancer Institute. Estimated Incidence and Mortality from Cancer in Brazil 2012.

Bagan JV, Scully C. Recent advances in Oral Oncology 2008; squamous cell carcinoma aetiopathogenesis and experimental studies. Oral Oncology. 2009; 45(6); 45-48.

Biazevic MGH, Antunes JLF, Castellanos-Fernandez RA, Michel- Crosato E. Trends in oral and oropharyngeal cancer mortality in the municipality of São Paulo, 1980-2002. Cad Saùde Pùblica. 2006; 22(2): 105-114.

Buss PM. Health promotion and quality of life. Ciência & Saùde Coletiva. 2000;5, (1):163-177.

Chaves SCL, Silva LMV. Oral health care and the decentralization of health in Brazil: A study of two exemplary cases in the state of Bahia. Caderno de Saùde Pùblica.

2007;23(5):1119-1131.

Cimard ACBS, Fernandes APS. Oral Cancer: The practice and clinical reality of dental surgeons in Santa Catarina. RFO. 2009;2(14):99-104.

Coelho MTAD, Almeida FILHO N. Conceitos de saùde em discursos contemporâneos de referência cientifica. História, Ciências, Saùde-Manguinhos, Rio de Janeiro. 2002;9(2):,315-333.

Costa JFR, Chagas LD, Silvestre RM, organizers. Brazil's national oral health policy: record of a historic achievement. Brasilia: Pan American Health Organization (PAHO); 2006.

Costa SM, Abreu MHNG, Vasconcelos M, Lima RCGS, Verdi M, Ferreira EF. Inequalities in the distribution of dental caries in Brazil: a bioethical approach. Cien Saude Colet 2013; 18(2):461-470.

Cruz GD, Le Geros RZ, Ostroff JS, Hay JL, Kenigsberg H, Franklin DM. Oral cancer knowledge, risk factors and characteristics of subjects in a large oral cancer screening program J Amer Dent Assoc. 2002;133(8):133 -138.

DGS. National Oral Health Program. Health risk assessment. Normative Circular No. 9= DSE of 19/07/2006. Lisbon. 2006.

Dedivitis RA, Epidemiologic clinical characteristics of squamous cell carcinoma of the mouth and oropharynx. Rev Odont Bras Central. 2004;70(1):35-40.

Department of Primary Care. Secretariat of Health Care, Ministry of Health. SB Brasil 2003 Project: oral health conditions of the Brazilian population 2002-2003. Main results. Brasilia: Ministry of Health; 2004.

Fejerskov O. Concepts of dental caries and their consequences for understanding the disease. Community Dent Oral Epidemiol.1997;25(1):5-12.

Copenhagen: Munksgaard; 1994;( )209-217.

Freysleben GR, Peres MAA, Marcenes W. Prevalence of caries and mean DMFT in schoolchildren aged twelve to thirteen in 1971 and 1997. Rev Saùde Pùblica. 2000; 34(3): 304- 308.

Gjermo P, Rosing CK, Susin C, Oppermann R. Periodontal diseases in central and south America.2002;29(1):70-78.

Goldbaum M. Epidemiology in health services. Cad Saùde Pùblica. 1996;12(2):95-98.

Goiato MC. Luciana C, Daniela MS, Humberto Filho G Wirley GA. Oral Injuries Caused by the Use of Removable Prostheses. Pesq Bras odontoped e Clin Integr. 200;5(1):85-90.

Gourin CG, Kaboli KC, Blumi EJ, Nance MA, Koch WM. Characteristics of participants in a free oral, head end neck cancer screening program. Laryngoscope. 2009;119(4):679-682.

Gushi LL, Soares MC, Forni TIB, Vieira V, Wada RS, Sousa MLR at al. Relationship between dental caries and socio-economic factors in adolescents. J Appl Oral Sci. 2005; 13(3):305-311.

National Cancer Institute. Cancer estimate 2016/2017. Available at http://www.inca.gov.br/estimativa/2016/estimativa-2016-v11.pdf. Accessed August 2016.

National Cancer Institute Available at http://www1.inca.gov.br/wcm/connect/tiposdecancer/site/home+/mouth/definition.

Accessed on March 9, 2018.

Jessor R, Bos JVD, Vanderry J, Costa FM, Turbin MS. Protective factors in adolescent problem behavior: moderator effects and developmental change. Developmental Psychology,Washington. 1995;31(6):923-933.

Lima AAS, França BHS, Ignàcio SA, Baioni CS. Knowledge of university students about oral cancer. Rev Bras Cancerologia. 2005;51(4):283-238.

Molina APS, Ribeiro MG, Silva JA, Torres-Pereira CC. Knowledge, practices and attitudes in relation to the diagnosis of mouth cancer in the view of the population. Revista Dens. nov/abril 2006;14(2):28 -33.

Mateus FO. Oral cancer in Brazil: Literature review.2008.

Marques DE, Rink MCM, Loureiro RMT, Silva VC. Epidemiological survey of dental caries in the rural area of Uberlândia, Minas Gerais; contribution to an oral health program model. Rev Cent Ciênc Bioméd Univ Fed Uberlândia. 1986;2(1):33-38.

Mauricio HA, Matos FCM, Guimarâes TMR. Knowledge, attitudes and practices about mouth cancer in the community served by the PSF in Sâo Sebastiâo do Umbuzeiro/PB. Rev. Bras. Cir. Head and Neck. 2009;8(1):10-14.

Massano J, Regateiro FS, Januârio G, Ferreira A. Oral squamous cell carcinoma: Review of prognostic and predictive factors. Oral Surg Oral Med Oral Pathol Oral Radiol Endod. 2006;102(1):67-76.

Minayo, MCS. Ecosystem approach to health and quality of life. In: Minayo, MCS;

Minayo, AC (Org.). Health and sustainable environment: Tightening the knots. Rio de Janeiro: Fiocruz, 2002; 173-189 Available from SciELO Books .

Neville BW, Damm DD, Allen CM, Jerry E. Pathologia Oral e Maxilofacial, 2 ed. Rio de Janeiro: Guanabara Koogan, 2004.

Neville BW, Damm DD, Allen CM, Chi AC. Oral and Maxillofacial Pathology, 4 ed. Rio de Janeiro: Guanabara Koogan, 2016.

Ogden GR. Alcohol and oral cancer. Alcohol. 2005;35(3): 163-169

Omena BD. Epidemiological survey of the need for dental treatment in rural schools in the municipality of Pindoba- AL. Federal University of Santa Catarina (TCC), 2016.

World Health Organization. Oral health epidemiological survey: instruction manual. Geneva; 1997.

Prado NF, Passarelli DHC. A new view on oral cancer prevention in the dental clinic. Rev.Odont.Univer. SP. 2009;21(1):29-85.

Pereira CP. Dentistry in collective health: planning actions and promoting health. Porto Alegre: Artmed; 2003.

Peres KGA, Bastos JRM, Latorre MRDO. Severity of tooth decay in children and relationship with social and behavioral aspects. Rev Saùde Pùblica. 2000; 34(4): 402-8.

Piemonte ED, Lazos JP, Brunotto M. Relationship between chronic trauma of the oral mucosa, oral potentially malignant disorders and oral cancer. Journal of Oral Pathology & Medicine. 2010;39(7): 513-517

Quirino MRS, Gomes FC, Marcones MS, Balducci I, Anbinder AL. evaluation of knowledge about mouth cancer among participants in a campaign for prevention and early diagnosis of the disease in Taubaté- SP. Rev. Odontol UNESP. 2006; 35(4):327-333.

Oral Health Epidemiological Survey Report. Village Paidéia module of the Barao Geraldo Health Center. Campinas: Municipal Health Department; 2003.

Ribeiro R, Martins MAT, Fernandes KPS, Bussadori SK, Miyagi SPH, Martins MD. Evaluation of the level of knowledge of a population regarding oral cancer. Robrac. 2008;17(4):194-199.

Roncali AG, Frazao P, Patussi MP, Araùjo IC, Ely HC, Batista SM. SB 2000 Project: a perspective for the consolidation of epidemiology in collective oral health. RBO. 2000;1(2):9-25.

Susser E.; Susser M. Choosing a future for epidemiology: II From Black Box to Chinese Boxes and Eco-epidemiology. American Journal of Public Health. 1996;86(5):674-677.

Starfield B. Primary care: balancing health needs, services and technologies. Brasilia:Unesco; Ministry of Health 2002.

Scheufen RC, Almeida FCS, Silva DP. Prevention and early detection of oral cancer: Screening in populations at risk. Pesq. Bras. Odontoped Clin. Integr. 2011;11(2):245-249.

Thylstrup A. When is caries, and what should we do about it? Quintessence Int 1998;29(9):594-597.

Tescarollo A, Freire D. Oral cancer: Brazil fails to save lives due to late diagnosis. Jorn sit odont. 2018.

Vidal AKL, Tenòrio APS, Brito BHG, Oliveira TBT. Pessoa, ID. Knowledge of schoolchildren in the Pernambuco Sertao about mouth cancer. Pesq Bras Odontoped Clin Integr, 2009; 9(3):283-288.

Wünsch-Filho V. The epidemiology of oral and pharynx cancer in Brazil. Oral Oncol.2002; 38:737-746.

Zain RB. Cultural and dietary risk factors of oral cancer and precancer a brief overview. Oral oncology. 2001, 37:205-210.

Zanetti F, Azevedo MLC, Perez DEC , Silva RSC. Knowledge and risk factors of oral cancer in a prevention program for truck drivers. Odontol Clin Cient. 2011;10(3): 233-241.

37

ANNEX A

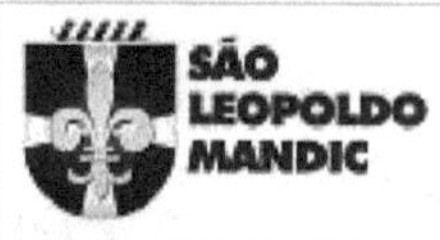 **FACULDADE SÃO LEOPOLDO MANDIC** 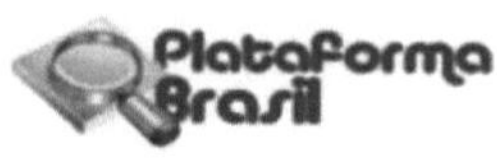

RESEARCH PROJECT DATA

Research Title: Epidemiological Survey of Risk of Dental Diseases, Need for Prosthesis Use and Active Search for Oral Cancer in the Municipality of Penedo- Alagoas

Researcher: EDILAINE SOARES DOS SANTOS

Thematic Area:

Version: 1

CAAE: 68611617.9.0000.5374

Proposing Institution: Centro de Pos-Graduagao Sao Leopoldo MandicZFaculdade de

Main Sponsor: Own Financing

OPINION DATA

Opinion Number: 2.115.933

Project presentation:

Epidemiological surveys are important for understanding the prevalence of oral diseases and thus planning, implementing and evaluating health actions, as well as identifying the treatment needs of a given population at a given time and place. In this way, this study will verify the prevalence of tooth decay, periodontal disease, active search for oral cancer, the need to use prostheses among different age groups and measure the need for oral health care, actions and promotion in different areas assisted by the Family Health Strategy in the municipality of Penedo-AL. This is a cross-sectional study with residents of rural and urban locations in the 0-2, 2-9, 10-19, 2059 and +60 age groups, classified by 9 dentists, previously trained and calibrated, as to their risk of caries: 1(low); 2(medium); 3{high}; periodontal disease (gingivitis, supporting tissues and periodontal alterations); oral cancer (marking areas of alteration in the mucosa, use of dental prostheses, habits and addictions) and the need to use maxillary and mandibular prostheses (yes or no). Analysis of the data will allow us to understand the local reality and the community in the urban and rural areas, which in turn will allow us to assess the effectiveness of oral health promotion and prevention measures, priority in care and access to dental services. The results will be subjected to the appropriate statistical tests for each situation, taking into account the level of significance.

Endereço: Rua José Rocha Junqueira Nº13
Bairro: Swift   **CEP:** 13.045-755
UF: SP   **Município:** CAMPINAS
Telefone: (19)3518-3601   **Fax:** (19)3211-3600   **E-mail:** cep@slmandic.edu.br

FACULDADE SÃO LEOPOLDO MANDIC

Significance of 5%.

Research Objective:

To demonstrate the importance of the epidemiological survey in the Oral Health Strategy based on the risk index, periodontal disease, contributing factors to the development of soft tissue lesions, the need for the use of dental prostheses and the knowledge of the conditions of different areas of the same municipality, in order to draw up a program of prioritization of care, control, promotion and prevention based on the profile of this population.

Evaluation of Risks and Benefits:

This study poses no risk to patients, as it is an observational study.

Comments and Considerations on the Research:

Not applicable.

Considerations on Mandatory Terms of Presentation:

All documents have been submitted and are duly completed.

Recommendations:

Not applicable.

Conclusions or Pending Issues and List of Inadequacies:

The project is suitable and ready for execution.

Final considerations at the discretion of the CEP:

The researcher should be aware that the research project approved by this CEP refers to the protocol submitted for evaluation, and is exempt from co-responsibility for research already carried out. Therefore, according to CNS Resolution 466/12, the researcher is responsible for "developing the project as outlined", and if there are any changes to this project, this CEP must be notified in an amendment via Piataforma Brasil, for a new evaluation.

This opinion is based on the documents listed below:

Document Type	Archive	Post	Author	Situation
Basic Project Information	PBASICINFORMATIONFROMPROJECT 925054.pdf	19/05/2017 17:02:38		Accepted
Cover Sheet	sheet.pdf	19/05/2017 17:01:00	EDILAINE SOARES DOS SANTOS	Accepted
Detailed Design	project.doc	19/05/2017	EDILAINE SOARES	Accepted

Endereço: Rua José Rocha Junqueira Nº13
Bairro: Swift   **CEP:** 13.045-755
UF: SP   **Município:** CAMPINAS
Telefone: (19)3518-3601   **Fax:** (19)3211-3600   **E-mail:** cep@slmandic.edu.br

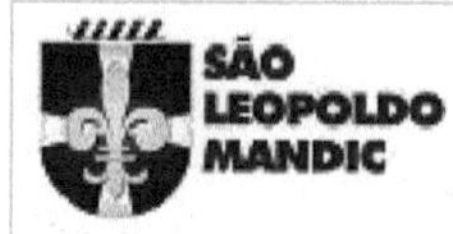

FACULDADE SÃO LEOPOLDO MANDIC

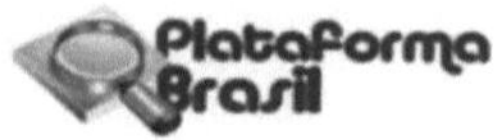

! Investor Brochure	project.doc		14:56:53	DOS SANTOS	Accepted
ICF / Terms of Assent / Justification for Absence	TCLE.docx		19/05/2017 14:54:01	EDILAINE SOARES DOS SANTOS	Accepted

Status of Opinion:

Approved

Needs CONEP appraisal:

No

CAMPINAS, June 12, 2017

Signed by:

Cecilia Pedroso Turssi

(Coordinator)

ANNEX B

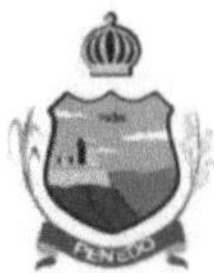 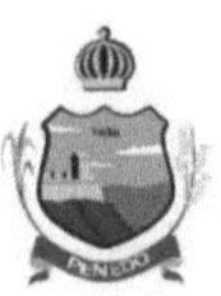

Penedo City Hall

Municipal Health Department Buccal

Health Coordination

TERM OF FREE AND INFORMED CONSENT (TCLE)

Penedo, 20 _________________________________. You are being invited as a

You are invited to take part in the **"Epidemiological Survey of Dental Disease Risk, Need for Prosthesis Use and Active Search for Oral Cancer"** research. In this research we intend to verify the prevalence of caries, periodontal disease, soft tissue alterations and the need to use prostheses, among different age groups in the population and to dimension the needs for assistance, actions and promotion in oral health in different areas assisted by the Family Health Strategy of the Municipality of Penedo-AL. The following procedures will be adopted for this study: The dental surgeon in the micro-area will carry out an intraoral examination at the individual's home, which will allow data to be collected to determine the individual's risk of dental caries, the presence of gum/periodontal disease, the presence of soft tissue erosion and the need to use dental prostheses, which will be recorded by the oral health assistant on a form standardized by the Alagoas State Secretariat, immediately after the examination. All the diagnostic criteria recommended by the WHO will be followed. All the necessary equipment will be used, namely gloves, masks and wooden spatulas. The tests will be carried out at room temperature.

The research poses no risk and will contribute to "Direct or indirect research benefits for participants". You will not receive any financial advantage for taking part in this study. You will be informed about the study in any way you wish and you will be free to participate or refuse to participate at any time and without any prejudice, and you will be able to withdraw from the study as soon as it is formalized. Your participation is voluntary and refusing to take part will not lead to any penalty or change in the way you are treated by the researcher, who will treat your identity with professional standards of confidentiality. The results of the research will be made available to you when it is finished. Your name or any other form that may indicate your participation will not be released without your permission.

You will not be identified in any publication that may result. The Researchers will treat your identity with professional standards of confidentiality, in compliance with Brazilian legislation (Resolutions n≡ 466/12; 441/11 and Ordinance 2.201 of the National Health Council and its Complementaries), using the seed information for academic and scientific purposes.

I, , bearer of the identity document, have been informed of the objectives of the research **"Epidemiological Survey of Risk of Dental Diseases, Need for the Use of**

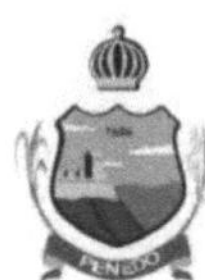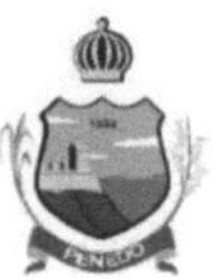

Prosthetics and Active Search for Oral Cancer", in a clear and detailed manner and I have clarified my questions.

questions. I know that at any time I can request new information and change my decision to participate if I wish.

I declare that I agree to take part in this research. I have received an original copy of this informed consent form and have been given the opportunity to read it and clarify my doubts.

Name	Participant's signature	Date
Name	Researcher's signature	Date

If you have any questions about the ethical aspects of this research, please contact us:

CEP - Ethics Committee Faculdade Sao Leopoldo Mandic

Rua José Rocha Junqueira, 13

13045-755 Campinas/SP

Phone:(19) 32113600

cep(5)slmandic.edu.br

Name of Researcher Responsible: Edilaine Soares dos Santos

Address: Conjunto Monte Rei, quadra B, n≡ 247, Penedo - Alagoas

Phone: 55(82)99922 5213

E-mail: Edilaine ssoares(⅞hotmail.com

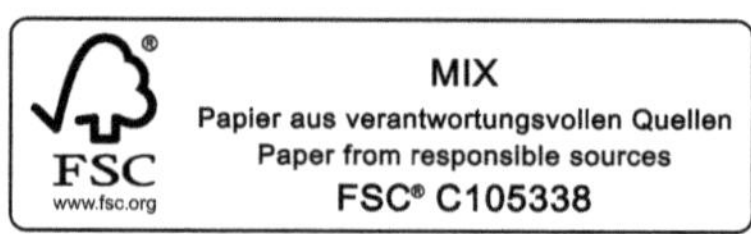

Printed by Books on Demand GmbH, Norderstedt / Germany